Relaxation and Exercise for the Childbearing Year

Eileen Brayshaw
MCSP, SRP, FETC

and

Pauline Wright
MCSP, SRP, FETC

Haigh & Hochland Publications Ltd
in conjunction with
The Royal College of Midwives

Published by Haigh & Hochland Publications Limited, 174a Ashley Road, Hale, Cheshire, WA15 9SF, England.

© 1996, Eileen Brayshaw and Pauline Wright
First edition

ISBN 1-898507-29-5

British Library Cataloguing in Publication Data
A catalogue record for this book is available from the British Library

Printed in Great Britain

Contents

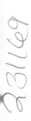

Acknowledgements

We would like to thank Jeanne McIntosh and Barbara LeRoy, Des, Sue and Jo for their invaluable help with the text and Janice Martin for the illustrations.

Introduction

Welcome to your childbearing year.

This book has been written for all of you who are pregnant or have recently given birth. It is in response to requests from women who want a reminder of the relaxation and exercises they have learned at antenatal classes, and also in response to the many midwives who have asked us for a comprehensive, yet simple book they can recommend to women asking for practical advice and skills for the childbearing year. Because we are both obstetric physiotherapists, we have not only the expertise in relaxation and exercise, but also in the knowledge of anatomical and physiological aspects of pregnancy and labour.

Many body changes take place during the childbearing year, and sometimes these can lead to long-term problems such as backache or stress incontinence. Most of these can be avoided by looking after your body in pregnancy and making sure you get back to normal quickly after the birth. This comprehensive, illustrated guide will help you to take care of your body through pregnancy, labour and afterwards. For those of you who are attending antenatal preparation classes, it will be a useful reminder of the exercises, relaxation and coping skills you are learning for labour and will allow you to practise these at home. For those of you who have not been taught these skills, this book describes them simply so you will be able to work through them with your partner. The last section is devoted to the postnatal exercises that are safe and effective to perform from the day of delivery up to three months afterwards and will prepare your body to resume more strenuous activities from then on. There are also sections dealing with some of the physical problems that occasionally arise during pregnancy and the postnatal period.

In the text we have referred to the birthing partner as 'he' and the midwife as 'she'. This is merely for ease of reference.

We hope you enjoy the book and we wish you all the best throughout your childbearing year.

SECTION ONE

Pregnancy

Now that you are pregnant you will be wanting to look after your body so you will feel fitter, be prepared for labour and get your figure back afterwards. Changes are happening in your body due to pregnancy hormones, so it is important that you choose safe but effective exercises for your fitness programme.

The exercises in this book have been carefully chosen with this in mind, but you must always work at your own pace and listen to your own body. If you have any problems in your pregnancy, ask your doctor's advice before starting any exercise programme.

If you are attending antenatal classes at your local hospital, health centre or the National Childbirth Trust, you may be practising some of the exercises and relaxation already. However, some classes do not start until after 30 weeks of pregnancy, and it is beneficial to start exercising earlier in your pregnancy.

Relaxation and exercise can help you to:
* feel more confident and have an improved self-image;
* improve muscle tone and flexibility for pregnancy and labour;
* lessen physical and emotional tension;
* improve posture and reduce backache;
* ease minor discomforts;
* sleep better;
* recover more quickly after your baby's birth;
* avoid long-term problems, e.g. backache and incontinence.

Antenatal exercise programme

If any exercises cause you discomfort, don't continue with them. If you are unsure about any of the exercises, ask your obstetric physiotherapist or midwife for guidance.

After about 20 weeks of pregnancy, it is not advisable to lie flat on your back to exercise. The weight of your uterus (womb) and growing baby press on blood vessels in this position and could interfere with your circulation. This is known as supine hypotension. You may feel faint and dizzy, and blood flow to the baby could be affected. Also avoid resting and sleeping flat on your back after about 20 weeks (see p.13 for alternative positions).

Circulatory exercises

Your circulation will be slower now because you have an increased blood volume and the walls of the blood vessels are more relaxed. As the baby and uterus grow, there will be extra pressure on your vessels and you might suffer from swollen ankles, cramp and varicose veins. To help avoid or relieve these problems, try the following.

Foot exercises

Sit on the bed, floor or chair with your legs straight and supported and your feet a few inches apart.

*   Bend and stretch your ankles briskly for at least half a minute.
*   Keeping your knees and hips still, circle both feet in as large a circle as you can for at least half a minute, changing direction halfway through.

Do these movements whenever possible – especially first thing in the morning and last thing at night.

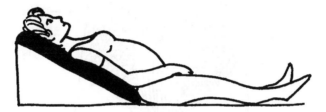

Fig. 1.1: Foot exercises

*   Avoid wearing anything tight or constricting on your legs, although support tights might be recommended. If they are, put them on before you swing your legs over the edge of the bed or, alternatively, rest with your legs up for about 20 minutes before putting them on.
*   Avoid standing still – change your position frequently.
*   Exercise regularly – walking and swimming improve circulation.
*   Rest with your legs raised and supported whenever you can.
*   Wear comfortable and well-supporting footwear with medium to low heels.
*   Don't sit with your legs crossed.
*   Avoid pointing your feet and toes forcefully – you may get cramp.

From around 25 weeks of your pregnancy, if you have any swelling in your ankles, hands and face, have your blood pressure checked as it sometimes means that you and your baby need extra medical care.

Abdominal exercises

You have three pairs of abdominal muscles which criss-cross each side and are called the obliques and transversus. Two more muscles called the rectus muscles (recti) run down your abdomen on either side of the linea alba (the 'central seam' of connective tissue which holds the abdominal muscles together). This line often becomes pigmented and brown during pregnancy. Your abdominal (tummy) muscles will undergo considerable stretching as your pregnancy advances. They have to stretch both widthways and lengthways. If this is your first baby, your waistline could increase from about 66cm (26") to 112cm (44") and the length of your abdominal muscles from about 31cm (12") to 51cm (20"). In subsequent pregnancies these could increase even more.

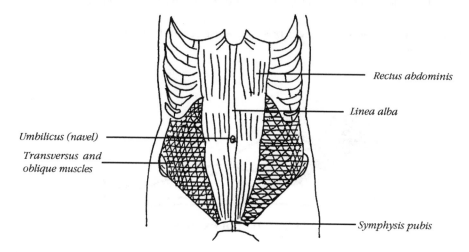

Fig. 1.2: Abdominal muscles

During pregnancy, hormones cause softening of the linea alba, making it more elastic. The growing uterus and baby stretch the abdominal muscles and linea alba and because of this, if posture is poor and the lower back is allowed to hollow too much, separation of the rectus muscles can occur. This separation is known as diastasis recti and once this has happened, strenuous abdominal work needs to be avoided because this may cause further separation and lead to long-term problems such as backache.

Your abdominal muscles support your back and growing baby and uterus. Now that the pregnancy hormones have softened your ligaments (strong bands of connective tissue which normally protect the joints), the muscles have to work extra hard to protect the joints of your pelvis and spine. Appropriate exercises are needed to maintain the strength and tone of the abdominal muscles:

Tummy-tightening

This is an easy exercise which you can practise often. Sit comfortably on a chair with your back and head supported and feet flat on the floor.

- Breathe in, breathe out, tighten your tummy muscles and pull the lower part of your tummy in towards your spine. Hold whilst you count to four, breathing normally. Repeat up to ten times, increasing the length of time you hold your tummy in if you feel comfortable.

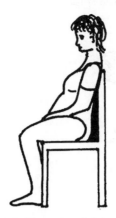

Fig. 1.3: Tummy tightening

Feel your abdominal muscles working. Practise this often in any position but **not** flat on your back after 20 weeks.

Pelvic tilting

Lie with your head and shoulders well supported by several pillows and a wedge or bean bag too if you have one. Bend your knees up and put your feet flat (see p.6).

- Pull in your tummy muscles, tighten the muscles of your buttocks and press the small of your back into the support. Hold this position for up to four seconds, breathing normally, then relax. Repeat five times and then gradually increase to ten if you feel comfortable.

Check that you are working your abdominal muscles, not just your buttocks! Once you have mastered the pelvic tilting exercise, you can try it at any time during your pregnancy in several other positions:

- sitting;

- reverse sitting;

- lying on your side;

- standing against a wall;

- standing sideways looking into a mirror – check your posture too!

- supported kneeling;

- on all-fours;

but **not** flat on your back after 20 weeks.

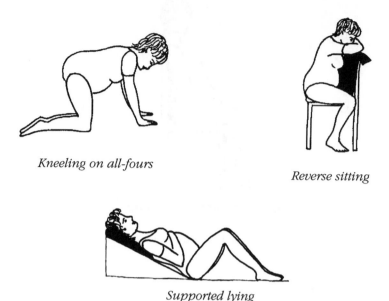

Kneeling on all-fours

Reverse sitting

Supported lying

Fig. 1.4: Positions for pelvic tilting

If pelvic tilting is done on all-fours, the abdominal muscles have to work harder against the downward pull of gravity. Ask your partner to check that you're not allowing your spine to sag or hollow, putting stress on the lower back. All-fours may not be a suitable position to use if you have Carpal Tunnel Syndrome (see p.27) as it can increase the discomfort in your hands and wrists.

Pelvic tilting may be performed rhythmically to relieve tension if you get postural backache.

Straight curl-up

Note that the curl-up exercise should only be done if you can hold your tummy flat throughout. This exercise should not be done after 20 weeks of pregnancy but discontinue it before then if any 'peaking or doming' occurs. Continuation could put stress on the area and increase diastasis of the rectus muscles (see p.4). Lie on your back with one pillow under your head and your hands on your thighs. Bend your knees up and put your feet flat.

- Pull in your tummy muscles, tighten the muscles of your buttocks and press the small of your back down on to the support (pelvic tilt). Hold this position whilst lifting your head and shoulders forwards and sliding your hands towards your knees. **Your tummy muscles must remain flat – there should be no 'peaking or doming'**. Breathe normally, then slowly lower your shoulders and head back on to the pillow before relaxing your pelvic tilt. Repeat five times increasing to ten if you feel comfortable – resting halfway if you need to.

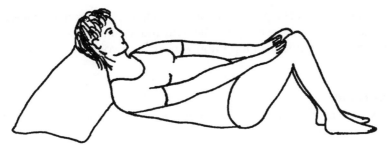

Fig. 1.5: Straight curl-up

Pelvic floor exercises

The pelvic floor is a sling or hammock of muscles forming the floor of your pelvis. It is attached to your tail bone at the base of the spine and to the pubic bone at the front of your pelvis. There are two layers of muscles with connective tissue between. Outlets from the bladder, uterus and bowel pass through the muscle layers. These outlets are known as the urethra, vagina and anus respectively. The muscle fibres form a ring around the anus and loop round the vagina and urethra forming a figure-of-eight.

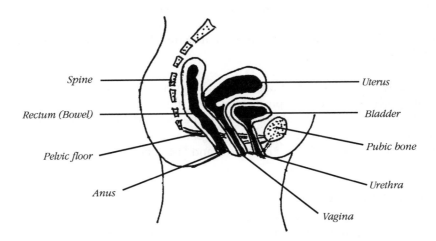

Fig. 1.6: Pelvic floor muscles

The pelvic floor supports the organs of the pelvis and holds everything in place. Action of the muscles helps to prevent leakage from the openings. Strong muscles contribute to the enjoyment of sex for both you and your partner. Your pelvic floor is under extra strain during pregnancy, carrying the added weight of your baby, and is also made more pliable by hormones. This allows the perineum (the area between the vagina and anus) to thin out and stretch more easily during delivery.

Pelvic floor exercises will help maintain tone and improve your control of these muscles. They should then relax more easily for the birth and regain their strength more quickly post-delivery. This should be a top priority exercise in your programme.

The exercise

Try the exercise in any comfortable position – but have your legs slightly apart and the rest of your body relaxed.

- Close your back passage as though you are stopping wind, close your middle and front passages too, as though stopping the flow of urine. Squeeze and lift up all three passages inside. Hold strongly for a few seconds, breathing normally throughout. Relax slowly and rest for a few seconds. Repeat the exercise slowly a few times.

Do this without pulling in your tummy or tightening your buttocks. Gradually increase the number of repetitions up to a maximum of ten and hold for up to ten seconds.

To check your pelvic floor muscles, try stopping the flow of urine mid-stream **occasionally** – but not if you have a urinary infection. Practice your pelvic floor exercise several times each day. Link it to something you do often, e.g. washing up, and try it after you have emptied your bladder. You may even stick coloured dots around the house to remind you! Make sure each tightening and hold is strong – better a few strong exercises than several weak ones! As your pregnancy progresses, this exercise may become more difficult and you may find the muscles tire more quickly at the end of the day.

When you feel really confident about the slow exercise, try up to ten slightly faster tightenings at the end of every practice session. These will help train your muscles to respond quickly to prevent leakage of urine when you cough, sneeze or even laugh! Always 'brace' (tighten) your pelvic floor **before** you cough, sneeze, laugh or lift an object and remember to practise both slow and fast tightenings.

Stretching exercises

These exercises will help prepare you both physically and psychologically to use a variety of positions during labour and delivery. You will learn to stretch and relax the muscles governing your joints. It may be best to avoid the squatting position if you have vulval varicose veins or haemorrhoids (piles) or if you have had a cervical suture. If you are concerned, check with your doctor or midwife before you start any of these exercises.

Always perform some warm-up exercises before you stretch, and **never** overstretch. Your ligaments are more elastic because of the effect of pregnancy hormones and if overstretched, could lead to unstable joints in the future. Your warm-up could include circulation exercises, bending and stretching alternate knees, pelvic tilting and walking. Perform the stretches slowly and breathe easily throughout.

Calf stretch

Stand at arms' length from a wall (not a door) with your palms pressed against it, and your left foot behind the right.

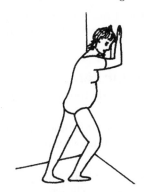

Fig. 1.7: Calf stretch

- Pelvic tilt – lean gently towards the wall bending your right knee and both elbows slightly. You should feel a stretch in your left calf muscles. Hold the stretch for up to ten seconds then relax. Change position and repeat, putting your right leg behind the left one.

If this feels very easy, move your back leg slightly further behind the front leg. Remember to keep your heels on the floor.

Inner thigh stretch

Do not do this if it causes any discomfort.

Sit on the floor with your back supported and the soles of your feet together, hands holding your ankles and feet pulled in towards your pelvis.

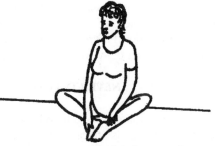

- Allow the weight of your legs to take your knees down towards the floor. Hold for up to ten seconds.

Fig. 1.8: Inner thigh stretch

Squatting

Do not do this if it causes any discomfort and never do it without plenty of support.

Hold on to a firm support or your partner, with your back straight and your feet and legs apart.

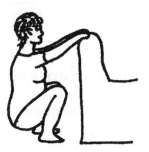

- Bend your knees so you are in a squatting position and hold the position for a few seconds and increase gradually to about one minute.

Fig. 1.9: Squatting

If you find this difficult, try placing one or two firm cushions or large books under your buttocks. Remove these one by one as your squatting improves.

Tailor sitting

Do not do this if it causes discomfort.

This is a stretching position which you can take up instead of sitting in a chair to read or watch television.

Sit on the floor with your back supported and the soles of your feet together, knees resting on pillows.

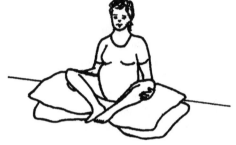

- Keep your feet close in to your pelvis, and hold this position for as long as you are comfortable.

Fig. 1.10: Tailor sitting

Follow your stretching exercises with some circulation exercises and pelvic tilts.

If you find the stretching exercises beneficial and want to try more, Yoga is recommended but do find an antenatal specialist. You may wish to exercise in a group, aquanatal and antenatal exercise-to-music are ideal, but do check that the instructor is a specialist antenatal teacher. Pregnancy isn't the time to take up new strenuous activity, but try swimming and a daily walk in the fresh air.

NEVER DO DOUBLE-LEG LIFTING OR SIT-UPS

Do discuss the safety and suitability of exercise/sport with an obstetric physiotherapist or specialist exercise tutor who teaches antenatal and postnatal women. Also, if you have any problems in your pregnancy, check with your midwife or doctor beforehand.

If in any doubt – check it out!

Back care, posture and lifting

As your pregnancy progresses and the weight and size of your baby increases, your centre of gravity moves forwards and upwards. You'll find you tend to tilt your pelvis further forwards than usual and your balance will alter. This can strain the ligaments and joints of your lower back and pelvis and could lead to discomfort, pain or fatigue. Your posture will depend on how strong your muscles are, the extra weight you've put on, how mobile your joints are and how tired you're feeling.

Good posture in all positions can help you to feel and look better as well as protecting your joints and preventing pain and discomfort.

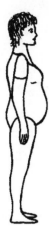

Fig. 1.11: Poor standing posture in pregnancy

Poor standing posture

- Poking chin

- Rounded shoulders

- Slack tummy muscles

- Hollow back

- Knees braced back

To correct your posture

Stand sideways to a long mirror and check your posture (preferably with little clothing on to allow your true silhouette to be seen).
- Put your feet apart, with your weight equally distributed on both legs.
- Relax your knees slightly.
- Tilt your pelvis by pulling in your tummy muscles, tightening the muscles of your buttocks and lessening the hollow in your back.
- Stand tall – imagine a string pulling up from the crown of your head.

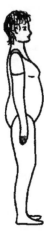

Fig. 1.12: Good standing posture in pregnancy

Good standing posture

- Chin tucked in

- Shoulders back and down

- Tummy muscles pulled in

- Back less hollow

- Knees slightly relaxed

- Have a look in the mirror and realign your body if you need to.

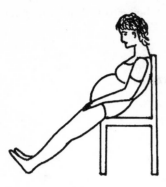

Poor sitting posture

- Poking chin

- Rounded shoulders

- Slouched body

- Thighs unsupported

- Feet resting on heels

Fig. 1.13: Poor posture in sitting

To correct your posture in sitting

Sit on a firm chair with your lower back supported – you may need a small cushion or rolled-up towel to achieve this. Your thighs should be supported by the chair with your feet should resting flat on the floor – use a small stool or cushion under your feet if you need to.

- Lift your ribs away from your hips so your chest is out and open, making more room for your baby.
- Lower your shoulders down and back.
- Tuck your chin in slightly.
- Imagine a string pulling the crown of your head upwards so you are sitting tall.
- Breathe easily.

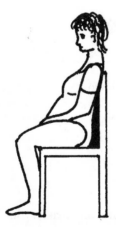

Good posture in sitting

- Chin tucked in

- Shoulders down and back

- Back supported

- Thighs supported

- Feet flat

A chair with a high back will support your head and shoulders and could be used for relaxation practice – even better if the chair has arms and if you can rest your legs on a stool or chair too. A firmer dining room-type may be more supportive and create a better posture than your soft, easy chair.

Fig. 1.14: Good posture in sitting

Lying postures

It's best not to lie flat on your back from about 20 weeks of pregnancy onwards because of the risk of supine hypotension (see p. 2). We all move around in bed when we're asleep, so you may wake up on your back – don't worry – just turn over again on to your side. Early in your pregnancy, if you choose to lie flat on your back, a pillow under your thighs may add to your comfort. As your body increases in size and weight, you will probably find it more difficult to get comfortable. Try a position which is well-supported and gives equal pressure on all parts of your body so you can rest and get some sleep.

SIDE-LYING

Lie on your side using two pillows under your head and one between your legs to help prevent strain on your pelvic joints. You may need a small cushion (or roll up the duvet) to support your abdominal muscles and your baby and another to support your forearm. If you have pain in your symphysis pubis (the joint at the front of your pelvis just below your baby), only use a very thin pillow or folded towel between your legs.

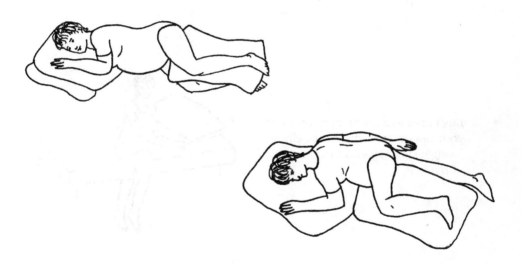

Fig 1.15: Side-lying and three-quarters lying

THREE-QUARTERS LYING

If you prefer to lie on your side with your underneath arm behind you, rest your head on one pillow and bring your top leg forwards and rest it on another pillow.

If you really can't get comfortable on your side, lie on your back with extra pillows and/or a wedge or bean bag to raise your head, shoulders and upper back. Another pillow, pulled well up under your thighs, will prevent the stretch on your lower back and knees.

When changing position in bed, bend your knees up and keep them pressed together. Roll over keeping your shoulders and knees in line – don't twist. Turning over in this way will protect your back, pelvic joints and abdominal muscles.

Getting up from lying in bed

Avoid sitting straight up forwards from lying as this risks straining your back and abdominal muscles. Instead:

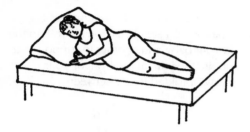

- bend your knees up and keep them together;
- roll your whole body over to one side – don't twist;

- push up into a sitting position using your upper hand and lower elbow, swinging your legs now over the side of the bed;

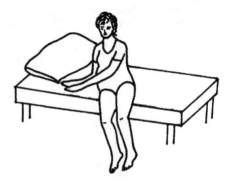

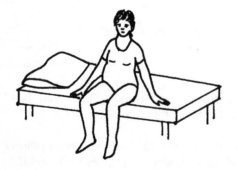

- sit on the side of the bed for a moment;
- stand up slowly, straightening your legs.

Do this in reverse when getting into bed.

Fig. 1.16: Getting up from lying in bed

Getting up from lying on the floor

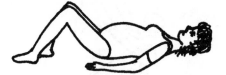

• Bend your knees up and keep them together;

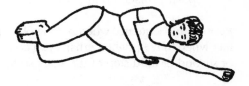

• roll over on to your hands and knees without twisting;

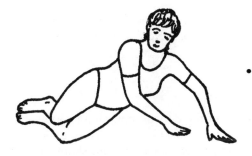

• come up to kneeling;

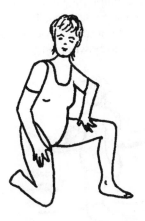

• bend one knee up;
• push yourself up, pressing your hands on to the thigh of your bent knee, slowly straightening your legs into the standing position.

Do this in reverse to get down on to the floor.

Fig. 1.17: Getting up from lying on the floor

Lifting

Avoid difficult heavy lifting during your pregnancy. If you have to lift (your toddler or basket of washing, for example):

- stand with your feet apart – one foot in front of the other;
- bend your hips and knees, keeping your back fairly straight;
- pull in your tummy and brace your pelvic floor;
- hold whatever you are lifting close to your body;
- push yourself up into standing.

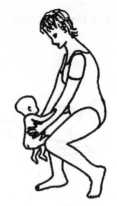

Fig. 1.18: Correct lifting technique

Reverse this sequence when putting objects down. Avoid twisting and only move your feet when fully upright. Perhaps you could encourage your toddler to stand on a chair or second or third step of the stairs so that you can avoid stooping when lifting.

Daily activities

The ligaments in your body have been softened by pregnancy hormones, especially those around your pelvis (ready for your baby's birth). So you need to protect all your joints when carrying out your daily activities.

In the home

Ask your partner or friend to help with some of the difficult household chores, e.g. moving furniture. Check the height of your working surfaces – you can't have a kitchen refit, but a few changes in working habits can prevent stress on your shoulders and back. For example, a high stool could prevent you leaning over too much, so try sitting to do some tasks such as food preparation. If you are short in stature, use the sink as a working surface for mixing bowls. If you are tall, try putting something under the washing-up bowl or under equipment on the working top to raise them up.

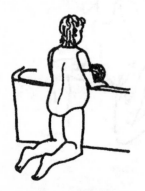

Fig. 1.19: Bathing toddlers

It takes practice to iron sitting down with the ironing board lower, but it will be less tiring than standing. If you do prefer to stand, make sure the ironing board is at the right height so you don't lean over too much. Have your feet apart so you can move your weight rhythmically from side to side.

Kneel or squat if you are reaching into low cupboards or doing gardening. Kneeling could also prevent backache when bathing your toddler, cleaning the bath or making the bed.

If vacuuming or mopping the floor, do it in a straight line and avoid twisting, as this could strain your pelvic joints.

Do plan with your partner the best way of caring for your baby in relation to safety and protection of both your backs. Think about what could be a problem, e.g. where to feed, change and bath baby and the suitability of baby equipment. This will help prevent unnecessary pain, discomfort and fatigue in the future.

Travelling

When getting into a car, sit on the seat first, tighten your tummy muscles (pulling your baby in) and keeping your knees together, bring your legs round into the car. Do this in reverse when getting out – think how a model does it! Avoid twisting round in a jerky way when putting the seatbelt on or if you have to reverse. Carry a small cushion, towel or cardigan to place behind your back during any journey, e.g. car, bus, train. Try to plan frequent stops to allow you to stretch your legs and back. You can use your pelvic tilting exercise to ease tension during the journey.

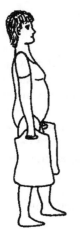

Shopping

When you are shopping, keep the supermarket trolley close to your body. If you haven't much shopping, try using the type designed for the elderly as these are not as deep and you won't have to lean over as far at the checkout. To carry shopping, either hold it close to your body, or divide the weight into equal amounts in each hand for balance and back care. If you've got a lot to carry, ask for help – many supermarkets employ staff to push trolleys or carry bags to the car.

Fig. 1.20: Carrying shopping

Working outside the home

If you have a standing job, check your posture and ease any discomfort with occasional rhythmical pelvic tilting. Help your circulation by moving around and sitting on a stool or chair when you can.

If you are sitting to work, think about your position. Your chair should give comfort and support. Do not assume that the chair that suited you before pregnancy fits you now you have changed shape. Can you alter the height of your chair? Have your work at a convenient level to prevent you having to lean forwards. If you have to sit most of the day, get up and walk around fairly often and do your pelvic tilting if you are uncomfortable.

Although you should not be doing heavy lifting during pregnancy, you may have to lift some objects. Be careful to do it correctly (see opposite).

Relaxation

Relaxation is a skill that you need to include in your exercise programme. It is not just lying or sitting still or napping in a dark, quiet room. Relaxation is recognizing and releasing the excess tension which can be present in our body whether we are active or at rest, thus reducing our overall body tension to a minimum. We should only use the muscles required for the job in hand and no more. Relaxation helps us to unwind from the stresses of everyday living. If practised daily during pregnancy, it gives opportunity for rest and conserves energy. Blood pressure will be lowered and some aches and pains relieved. We will cope better with pregnancy, feel less tired and have a feeling of well-being – your baby will enjoy it too! Once mastered, relaxation can be included as one of the coping strategies for labour and can be used after your baby is born, when life gets hectic and is exhausting. It will be a skill for life – your partner could benefit from learning it too!

We are all under pressure of some sort or another and most of us show signs of the stresses of modern day living. Coping with children, ageing parents, struggling round the shops, traffic and balancing work with home life are just a few examples. Pregnancy adds its own stresses on top of these.

Our bodies recognize when we're under stress by increasing certain hormones – including adrenaline, and preparing for 'fight or flight'. This is a primitive animal response – an emergency reaction. However, in humans this reaction is produced not just when there is real 'danger', but also when there is no real threat to life at all. Our bodies are unable to tell the difference between real and imaginary threats. We need some tension to perform and the occasional increase of hormones won't do much harm if, when appropriate action has been taken and the 'danger' is over, everything settles down to normal and relaxation takes place. But there is a problem when too many stressful situations follow each other and the reactions are continued. The result can lead to fatigue, pain and possible symptoms of illness such as raised blood pressure, headaches, insomnia and depression.

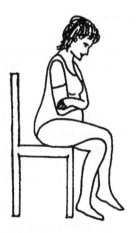

When under stress our bodies assume the common posture of tension:

- shoulders hunched;
- arms with elbows bent, close to body;
- hands clenched, gripping, finger-tapping;
- legs crossed, wound round chair leg;
- feet pulled up, tapping, walking round;
- body bent forward, stiff;
- head forward, jutting chin;
- face with jaw clenched, teeth grinding, frowning.

This posture of tension will be modified depending on the body's position, e.g. sitting, standing, lying.

Fig. 1.21: Posture of stress in sitting

The 'danger' message is received by our brain and internal responses are also made. The heart speeds up, blood pressure rises and breathing becomes rapid and shallow or the breath is held. Extra blood is sent to the brain, lungs and working muscles. Digestion slows down, we sweat more and our skin becomes clammy. The mouth becomes dry and the tongue sticks to the roof of the mouth.

Many of us take up a part of this posture of tension as a habit even when no stress is present. Indeed, even remembering previous pain, anger, worry, anxiety or frustration can give rise to these stress postures and responses.

If stress is prolonged, others will notice the signs of strain – grumbling, irritability, forgetfulness and inadequate sleep. If we go on like this, 'the straw will finally break the camel's back' – we can't cope and we break down.

Now that you are pregnant, you may be feeling physically exhausted and have aching joints. You may also have added worries and anxieties (as well as those mentioned above) regarding the baby, finances, returning to work after the baby's birth – and, of course, about labour and motherhood. There may be many more – in fact, pregnancy rates highly on a scale of various stressful events.

So how can you cope with stress?

- Breathe slowly and easily.
- Learn to understand yourself and how much you can put up with – if you can't cope, admit it and ask for help.
- Take time out – for hobbies and leisure activities, a walk outside or a warm bath.
- 'Create some space' for yourself if possible.
- Eat well, exercise and keep fit.

However you also need to recognize that relaxation can be a way of dealing with stress. A state of muscle relaxation is not compatible with that of anxiety – a relaxed person cannot be anxious, nor when anxious can a person be truly relaxed.

There are several relaxation techniques, and if you are already attending antenatal preparation sessions or Yoga, you may find that the one taught there works well for you. However, physiological relaxation is a simple and exact method widely taught and used by obstetric physiotherapists and midwives. The basis of this method is that when one group of muscles contracts (shortens) the opposite group of muscles relaxes (lengthens). Try this – make a fist with your hand, the muscles on the inside and palm (flexors) are contracting or shortening whilst the opposite group of muscles on the back of your hand and fingers (the extensors) are relaxing or lengthening. This reciprocal contraction and relaxation of opposing muscle groups has to occur to allow the movement of a joint to take place. So, to release the tension in your flexor muscles, stretch out your fingers and thumb like a fan. The extensors on the back of your hand and fingers are now contracting (shortening) and the opposite muscles on the front of your fingers and palm have had to relax (lengthen). Stop stretching out your fingers and thumb. Now neither group of muscles is working, resulting in a mid-position of the joints or position of ease. Confirmation of this comfortable position is sent to the brain from receptors in the joints and muscle tendons.

Posture of ease

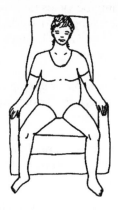

Fig. 1.22: Posture of ease in sitting

- Shoulders down.
- Arms with elbows slightly bent and a gap between elbows and body.
- Hands with fingers long and supported.
- Legs slightly apart, knees slightly bent.
- Feet pointing slightly away from face.
- Body supported if sitting or back-lying, slightly flexed if side-lying.
- Head in mid-position, supported if possible.
- Face with slack jaw, tongue resting low in the mouth, teeth slightly apart, no frown lines.

This posture of ease will be modified depending on the body's position, e.g. sitting astride a chair, lying, kneeling.

Relaxation technique

You need to give clear and concise instructions to each area of the body affected by stress. Three instructions are used in a definite sequence throughout the body. The result will be the position of ease and the brain will recognize and record this position. With practice, awareness of changing the position of tension to one of ease can be learned (like riding a bike), and will become automatic.

To move from the posture of tension to one of ease, the orders for each area of tension are:
1. **contract** the opposite muscle group strongly;
2. **stop** contracting that muscle group;
3. **be aware** of the resulting position of comfort.

The recommended sequence for the relaxation is:
- arms;
- legs;
- body;
- head;
- face;
- breathing.

Relaxation instructions

Sit well back in an armchair with your head supported, your arms and hands resting on the arms of the chair and feet flat on the floor. You may need a small cushion behind your back and another under your feet if they don't reach the floor.

ARMS

Shoulders
- Pull your shoulders down towards your feet.
- **Stop** pulling your shoulders down.
- Feel that your shoulders are now lower and your neck is longer.

Elbows
- Push your elbows slightly away from your side.
- **Stop** pushing your elbows out.
- Be aware that your elbows are open and slightly away from your side.

Hands
- Stretch out your hands, fingers and thumbs.
- **Stop** stretching them out.
- Note that your hands, fingers and thumbs are fully supported. Feel the surface on which they are resting.

LEGS

Hips
- Roll your hips and knees outwards.
- **Stop** rolling outwards.
- Be aware that your legs are slightly apart and turned away from each other.

Knees
- Adjust until comfortable.
- **Stop** adjusting.
- Reflect on the resulting position.

Feet
- Gently push your feet down, away from your face.
- **Stop** pushing them down.
- Feel your feet resting lightly on the floor.

BODY
- Press your body into the back of the chair.
- **Stop** pressing.
- Consider the sensation of your body resting against the support.

HEAD
- Press your head into the support.
- **Stop** pressing.
- Feel your heavy head resting comfortably against the support.

FACE

Jaw

- Keeping your lips closed, pull down your lower jaw.
- **Stop** pulling down.
- Feel that your teeth are no longer touching and that the jawline is slack.

Tongue

- Move your tongue low in your mouth.
- **Stop** moving.
- Register that your tongue is lying low in your mouth.

Eyes

- Close your eyes if you wish to, or stare instead.

Forehead

- Imagine someone smoothing away your frown lines from your eyebrows up over the top and the back of your head.
- Stop doing this.
- Feel the smoothing of the skin.

BREATHING

- Sigh out.
- Breathe low down in your chest at your own natural resting breathing rhythm with slight emphasis on the out breath.

You should gradually develop a pleasant feeling of comfort throughout your body. To prevent your brain being too active during your physical relaxation, concentrate on something pleasant and happy which is personal to you and which helps you to stay comfortable. Some women enjoy music in the background, but it needs to be relaxing – not with any beat. You may prefer to think about your breathing – natural, easy breathing at your own rate, low in your chest and concentrating on the relaxing outward breath. Notice the slight pause at the end of your outward breath before your inward breath follows automatically. This recognition of your own individual breathing rhythm is termed breathing awareness. The whole sequence of relaxation needs to be repeated just a little more quickly. Your birthing partner could help you to practise relaxation and also recognize your individual breathing rhythm so he can support you in labour.

This deep relaxation is often referred to as passive relaxation – where you are taking a break from the outside world. At the end of your period of relaxation, open your eyes and consider your position – how open and unfolded you are compared with the tense position of stress.

Do remember to move slowly following your relaxation. Stimulate your circulation by performing foot and hand movements before sitting forwards then standing up slowly. Try to practise this relaxation technique every day – perhaps whilst you're watching television either sitting in an armchair as before or with your legs up on a stool. Try it lying on the bed for an afternoon rest, or at night before going to sleep (see comfortable lying positions, p.13). You will need even longer time to 'come round' following relaxation in any lying position. Stimulate your circulation before slowly sitting up, then stretching and finally standing up. Remember to protect your back and tummy muscles as you get up by rolling on to your side (see p. 14). In your daily life try to be aware of the areas of your body which become tense most frequently – it is often shoulders, hands and face – check these in everyday situations and work into the position of ease.

Giving birth is probably the greatest athletic experience you are likely to take part in – both physically and emotionally. You may be apprehensive about labour. If you are delivering in hospital, tension may be increased by taking on a patient's role and by being in a different environment from home. You may feel you might not have responsibility for your own labour, or that you might lose control and dignity. In this respect, women vary enormously – labours are different too. Your partner may also have anxieties to a lesser degree.

The 'fight or flight' reaction is made in response to pain, fear or apprehension and can lead to increased physical discomfort and the slowing down of uterine activity and dilatation of the cervix.

With practice, relaxation can be used as a coping skill for labour. Energy will be conserved and your blood pressure kept lower by passive relaxation between contractions. A quicker relaxation needs to be used during contractions to increase your endurance to pain and allow labour to progress more easily. In order for you to be able to use the relaxation skill for labour, frequent practice is essential.

As well as relaxing in the comfortable positions described earlier (see p.31), you need to try out this skill using positions that you may adopt in labour. Ask your partner to try these out with you so he will be able to help you with the quick release of body tension. You should then be able to use relaxation together with breathing awareness during labour. At the start of a contraction, he will need to help you run through the sequence quickly to gain your position of ease rapidly. At the end of a contraction, he will need to check through with you to get the 'ripple effect' of relaxation spreading through your body to make use of the time between contractions to rest and conserve energy. As labour progresses, there will be less time to achieve this.

Relaxation can also help you to be more comfortable during a vaginal examination. Use your breathing awareness and relaxation especially allowing your mouth, jaw and pelvic floor to be slack.

Following delivery, do try to include relaxation in your daily routine. It is also a good coping skill for dealing with your baby. Not only should you feel less tired, but it can also be valuable if you are breastfeeding. You will be more comfortable and your milk will flow more easily. Your baby will be more relaxed too.

Touch
Simple touch is a means of contact giving reassurance and can be used to relieve tension. It can be practised during your pregnancy to give you another coping strategy for labour. Your birthing partner can learn to recognize any areas of tension in your

body and you will learn to respond to his touch. For example, ask your partner to place his hands gently but firmly on your shoulders – you should respond by relaxing the area beneath his hands. Together you can work out a plan for encouraging relaxation in the areas most likely to be tense.

Massage

For thousands of years, massage or 'the laying on of hands' has been used to heal and soothe. It is another means of giving physical contact, reassurance, warmth, pleasure and comfort. Massage involves stroking, kneading or pressure. It relieves pain by a diversionary effect and by stimulating the nerve endings in the skin which block some of the pain messages travelling to the brain. It encourages the release and circulation of endorphins (our own pain-relieving agents). It also helps to relax tense muscles. Massage improves the oxygenated blood supply to the area and removes lactic acid (waste products) which causes muscle aches. Those performing the massage gain a feeling of giving and participation.

Positions for massage

EXAMPLES

- Sitting astride a chair.
- Side-lying with pillows for support.
- Kneeling leaning forwards on to a support, i.e. where the back is exposed but the body is well-supported.

Although skin-to-skin contact is better, it can still be beneficial to massage through clothes.

Hints for the masseur

- Have warm relaxed hands. This will be more comfortable for your partner and you will be less likely to get cramp.
- Put a little baby oil or body lotion on your hands so that skin-to-skin contact doesn't cause friction.
- **If you are using aromatherapy oils it is essential that you seek expert advice on those suitable for use in pregnancy and labour (some are potentially dangerous).**
- Keep your movements slow – it's more relaxing.
- Don't be frightened of applying firm deep pressure when massaging her back – this is usually more comfortable than light pressure.
- Ask your partner for feedback on how it feels and whether it is in the right place.

Massage techniques

STROKING

Try long slow firm stroking down the length of her back. You can include the shoulder areas. Start in the middle, either side of the spine, and work outwards. Use each hand alternately so you always have one hand in contact with her back. In labour, your partner may also like firm stroking down her thighs.

KNEADING

Use one hand to support her pelvis and place your other flat on her back, relaxing your fingers. Make small deep circles moving the palm of your hand and her skin together over the underlying muscles – don't just rub over the surface of the skin. After a few circular movements in one area, move your hand gradually to another area. Provided your partner is well-supported, you can try doing this kneading with both hands.

PRESSURE

You can apply pressure to your partner's lower back using both hands. Place one hand on top of the other and apply pressure in time with her breathing. As she breathes in press firmly, as she breathes out release the pressure, but do not lose skin contact with your hands. When you are using this in pregnancy it should be in time with your partner's natural breathing rhythm. In labour you may be able to encourage slower breathing if your partner's breathing rate is too fast.

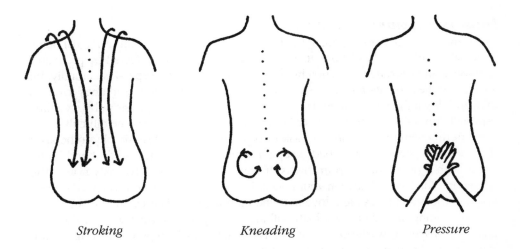

Stroking   *Kneading*   *Pressure*

Fig. 1.23: Massage techniques

Some physical problems in pregnancy

You will feel very pleased if you sail through your pregnancy without any complications, but you may experience some of the following physical problems which could make you feel miserable, uncomfortable or tired. If these problems can be relieved or overcome altogether, you will feel more relaxed and able to cope better.

Cramp

Cramp is very common during pregnancy and especially affects the calf muscles. Its cause isn't really known. The circulatory exercises can help in preventing attacks, so these need to be practised especially before sleep, as cramp often happens at night. Stretching the leg and pointing the foot down forcefully often causes cramp, so the feet need to be pulled up when having a stretch – it should become automatic eventually! To relieve calf cramp, the muscle can be put on the stretch by pulling the foot up until the pain subsides. Afterwards, massaging the calf muscles and briskly exercising the feet will improve comfort.

Varicose veins

Pregnancy hormones relax the vein walls and together with the increased pressure within the abdomen can cause varicose veins. Circulatory exercises should improve the flow of blood returning to the heart and sometimes, support tights are recommended. Prolonged standing and sitting with the feet down or legs crossed can aggravate the condition. The veins usually return to normal gradually after your baby is born.

Diastasis symphysis pubis

The symphysis pubis is the joint at the front of your pelvis – you can feel it just below your baby. This joint has ligaments which, like all others, are affected by pregnancy hormones and become more stretchy. In all women, the joint separates naturally, but sometimes the separation is excessive and leads to pain and acute tenderness over the joint and down the inner thighs. This is known as diastasis symphysis pubis. Walking, especially up stairs, and turning over in bed increase pain and become difficult. If you are suffering with these symptoms, ask to be referred to an obstetric physiotherapist. If the pain is severe, rest in bed, keeping your legs together, slightly bending the knees with a pillow under your thighs. If lying on your side, have only a very thin pillow or folded towel between your knees. To reduce the pain, you will need to bend up your knees and press them together when turning in bed and getting in and out of the car. Getting in and out of a bath will aggravate pain, so use a walk-in shower if possible, or have a wash-down instead. Try to take small steps when walking, and avoid stairs whenever possible. A supporting belt may be prescribed. Your doctor and midwife will need to be aware of your condition as you will need special help with positioning during labour and follow-up care by an obstetric physiotherapist is essential after delivery.

Carpal tunnel syndrome

About half of pregnant women have symptoms of this syndrome. It is caused by pressure on a nerve as it passes through a tunnel in front of the wrist bones. It usually starts after about 24 weeks of pregnancy. There could be numbness and stiffness of the fingers and possible difficulty in picking up and holding small objects, doing up buttons and other small movements. The problem seems worse in the morning and during the night when it can cause the sufferer to wake up. Wrist splints are often supplied to help give relief at night but can be worn during the day too. The hands and arms need to be supported on cushions or pillows when sitting and wrist and hand exercises may help. Doing these in cold water can give temporary relief. If you suffer from this condition, do take extra care when handling hot liquids, the kettle, teapot or cups especially first thing in the morning. Carrying heavy bags could make the symptoms worse. The condition usually clears up gradually following delivery of your baby.

Rib-pain (stitch)

Pregnant women often experience a stitch-like pain along the lower front and side ribs. It may be caused by the ribs flaring out, by the stretching of the abdominal muscles and by poor posture. Relief can often be felt by doing the following arm and side stretching.

ARM AND SIDE STRETCHING

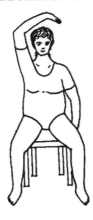

Fig. 1.24: Arm and side stretching

Sit upright on a stool with your feet flat on the floor and your left hand holding the seat.

* Slowly stretch your right arm above your head and bend your trunk very slightly to the left. Hold for a few seconds before lowering your arm down. Then stretch with your left arm.

Reverse-sitting astride a chair can be a comfortable position (see diagram p. 6).

Low back pain

Prevention of back pain is, of course, the ideal. However many pregnant women do suffer from this problem. If the pain is acute, the 'first aid' is bed rest in a comfortable position such as side-lying with a pillow between the legs. Comfort can often be gained by placing a hot water bottle wrapped in towels against the back. Referral to an obstetric physiotherapist for assessment and treatment is recommended where possible. When the pain is less severe, pelvic tilting can be tried and the advice on posture and back care needs to be followed and continued after the baby is born. Avoid any exercises which make the pain worse. A pelvic support may be prescribed for daytime use or a pantie-girdle could give some relief. Even if a support is worn, care should still be taken to protect the joints.

Stress incontinence

This is a leakage of urine on coughing, sneezing, lifting or even laughing. It is common during pregnancy especially during the last three months. Regular exercising of the pelvic floor muscles should help, but if the stress incontinence is severe antenatally, referral to an obstetric physiotherapist is advisable. The problem usually clears up after delivery of the baby but if not, an obstetric physiotherapist can assess and treat the condition.

Tiredness

Women often feel very tired during the first three months of pregnancy when so many changes are taking place. In the last three months, there is again tiredness as the baby has grown and the body is generally heavier. Ideally, workload needs to be cut down and partners asked to give more help with household tasks and looking after other children. Extra rest is essential and relaxation beneficial.

SECTION TWO

Labour

You may be attending classes run by a midwife or an obstetric physiotherapist and will have learnt about what happens in labour. However, if you are unable to get to classes, ask your midwife if there is anything you don't understand in the following section.

Labour has three stages. The **first** stage is the longest and you will have many contractions or shortenings of the muscles of your uterus (womb) with relaxation in between. The contractions pull up the cervix (neck of the womb) and gradually open it wide enough (about 10cm in diameter) for your baby to pass through.

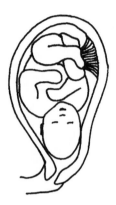 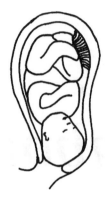 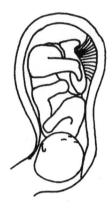

Fig. 2.1: Cervical dilatation

This is a passive stage for you and you can help most by letting nature get on with the job and not allowing yourself to become anxious or tense. However this isn't always easy because, although the contractions are mild and painless initially, they become stronger and painful as labour progresses and our usual response to pain is to tense up. This in turn makes the pain feel worse.

Certain skills may help you to cope with this stage and allow you to remain calm and conserve your energy for the hard work that the second stage of labour will bring. Practising these coping strategies with your birthing partner during pregnancy will help to increase your confidence.

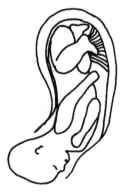

The **second** stage of labour is the passage of the baby from the uterus down the vagina (birth canal) once the cervix has dilated sufficiently and ends with the birth of your baby.

This is the stage where labour is really hard work, so you will be glad you didn't waste your energy during the first stage. You will be able to join in with the contractions of the uterus and help to push your baby out.

The **third** stage of labour is the delivery of the placenta (afterbirth) and involves the midwife more than you – you will be much more interested in looking at your baby!

Fig. 2.2: Second stage

Coping skills for the first stage of labour

Most of the skills which will help you to cope with the first stage of labour have been covered earlier in this book. However they need to be put together and some may need to be modified.

Early first stage

You may feel the very early contractions as slight backache or period-like pains and they are usually more uncomfortable than painful. Each contraction may last up to 40 seconds and be up to 30 minutes apart. If it is night-time, try to rest. During the day, you may prefer to carry on with everyday activities, have a light snack, relax in a warm bath or pass the time watching television.

The position you adopt during contractions should help you to stay calm and comfortable. Some positions also help labour to progress. Try different ones with your partner during pregnancy and practise the relaxation technique in each of the positions. If you feel the contractions in your back, try leaning forwards. Positions such as high-kneeling or kneeling on all-fours, reverse-sitting astride a chair, or just standing leaning forwards may be comfortable. Some of these positions also allow the joints of the pelvis to give a little, producing more space for baby's descent through the pelvis.

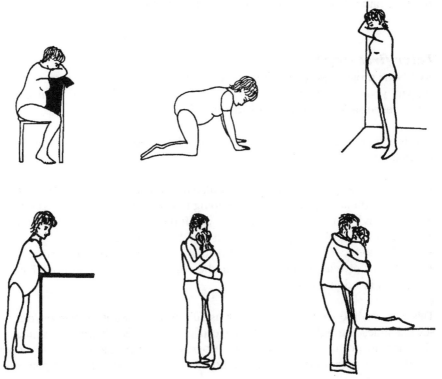

Fig. 2.3: Alternative positions for the first stage of labour

Other positions you may prefer are lying on your side, sitting well supported on the bed, on a beanbag or in a rocking chair. Some of these positions will allow your partner to massage your back, another way of coping with the discomfort (see p.24).

Because you have learnt about what happens to your body during labour, you should be less anxious and so less likely to tense up during the contractions. Pain and strong emotions also make us tense, so you will need to concentrate on your relaxation during the contractions to stay calm. Remember that tension uses up a lot of energy and valuable oxygen which is needed by your baby and by the muscles of the uterus so they can work strongly. The more you relax, the more easily your labour will progress.

The breathing awareness you performed at the end of your relaxation sequence (see p. 22) will help to keep your breathing at your own natural rate during the contractions and your partner should be quite accomplished at recognizing this by now. Remember that it is the outward breath that is the relaxing phase of breathing. Therefore just concentrate on each outward breath, appreciating the pause after it before you automatically breathe in again.

You will find it helps to have a positive attitude to your contractions as each one has its role to play. If this is acknowledged it will be easier to accept and to cope with them. Equally, you may find it helpful to tick off each contraction mentally as it finishes, rather like a milestone on the journey to full dilatation of the cervix.

Later first stage

As labour progresses, you will feel the need to pause when a contraction starts and prepare yourself for it. It is at this time that you will probably find you need a plan of action, especially if you haven't had any pain relief.

The following 'five point plan' summarizes all the skills you have been learning in pregnancy.

- First – be positive. Greet the contraction mentally – remember it is going to perform an important role in helping to open up the cervix to its full extent.
- Second – make sure you are in a comfortable position of ease (see p.31).
- Third – check that your shoulders and hands are relaxed.
- Fourth – concentrate on your breathing throughout the contraction.
- Fifth – give a big sigh of relief at the end of the contraction now that it is over and has done its job.

This is an outline which you may find useful. You may want to change your position several times throughout the first stage of labour. It has been shown that regular alteration in posture helps labour to progress. Your position will also depend on whether you have a drip and/or monitors in place and what form of pain relief you have chosen.

As labour progresses you may find yourself tightening up in an attempt to fight the pain. As already explained, this will only make things worse; your shoulders will tense up and your breathing may become quicker and shallower. If this 'panic' breathing continues for any length of time it could lead to hyperventilation or 'overbreathing'. This is a state where your body is getting too much oxygen and this can be just as dangerous as having too little. This could also affect your baby's oxygen levels, so it is a situation to be avoided. It could be said to be an SOS situation – one which will get worse if things aren't reversed. S, O and S are also the initials of an adapted breathing awareness which will help to prevent hyperventilation, i.e. **S**igh **O**ut **S**lowly. Try it now in front of a mirror. You will notice that, as well as your breathing slowing down to its natural rate, your shoulders will sag as you breathe out, allowing them to relax. The SOS breathing can be used during any of the first stage contractions if you prefer, rather than using your breathing awareness, and your partner can breathe with you. However, SOS can be helpful when the contractions are stronger and your partner may have noticed that you are tensing slightly. If you do actually hyperventilate, you may experience a tingling sensation in your hands and feet or down the side of your face, feel light-headed, clammy and have palpitations. The quickest way of dealing with this, is to cup your hands over your nose and mouth and breathe in and out into your hands. This way you will be breathing your own carbon dioxide back into your lungs and this will cancel out the excess oxygen induced by overbreathing.

End of first stage (transition)

Towards the end of the first stage of labour, the contractions are longer, stronger and closer together. They are really working hard at opening up the cervix. You may start to feel very frustrated and fed-up and may even blame your partner for everything. You might use strong language and tell your partner to leave. This is common behaviour that the staff all recognize as being part of this particular time in labour and usually means you are nearly ready for the second stage. Your midwife won't mind at all if you 'let off steam' verbally – it is another way of relieving tension and she will have seen and heard it all before!

When the cervix is fully dilated, your baby's head will move down slightly and you may feel pressure on to your bowel. This will give you the urge to push, and very often it is this sensation that is the sign that the end of the first stage has been reached and the hardest work is about to begin. Sometimes, however, this urge can be present before the cervix is completely dilated and it could prolong the first stage. Don't give in to this feeling until your midwife has given you the go ahead. You may have a few contractions where you have to stop yourself from pushing. It is the position of your baby's head which is causing the pressure and giving the premature urge to push, so you could alter your position to ease this sensation. Sitting upright will cause most pressure, but tilting to one side with pillows behind you or lying on one side will relieve some of that pressure. Kneeling on all-fours with your head resting on your hands will take away most of the unpleasant sensation, although this position is not always practical or comfortable at this time.

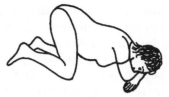

Fig. 2.4: Knee chest position to prevent pushing

Altering your breathing should also help. You will want to hold your breath and bear down; instead try to concentrate on breathing out in groups of three. Give two short sharp blow-breaths out followed by one longer blow out with a relaxed mouth, making a noise so your breath can be heard. This interrupted breathing will stop your diaphragm (a sheet of muscle which separates your chest from your abdominal cavity) pushing downwards and increasing the pressure within your abdomen. You can call it 'puff-puff-blow' or whatever you prefer. The main thing to remember is that the three breaths all occur on one outward breath, don't breathe in between them. This will require your concentration and will help to take your mind off the desire to push. Practise this breathing with your partner, you may not have to use it, but it is useful to know 'just in case'. If you do need to use this in labour, it works best if your birthing partner takes the lead and you follow, keeping eye contact throughout the contraction.

Second stage

The position you adopt for the contractions of the second stage can assist the passage of your baby along the birth canal. Remember, if you are lying on your back it is an uphill struggle. Squatting is the optimum position where gravity is assisting and your pelvis is at its widest. This requires preparation, practice and a lot of support from your partner. Many women are not comfortable with this if it is not a position they normally adopt.

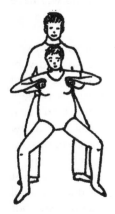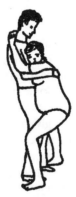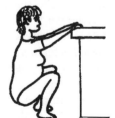

Fig. 2.5: Squatting for second stage

Variations on squatting, e.g. supported on a beanbag or cushions may be more acceptable. Kneeling almost upright supported by your partner, or kneeling on all-fours are easier positions to maintain, yet still advantageous.

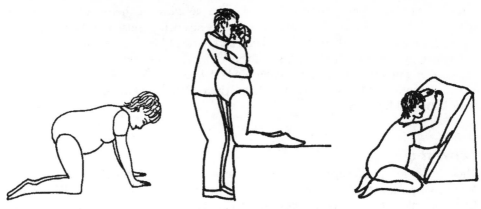

Fig. 2.6: Kneeling for second stage

Most women find that sitting upright and well-supported suits them, but make sure you don't slip down too far during the contractions and end up lying on your back or you will find it difficult to push.

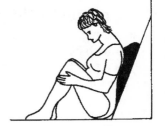

Fig. 2.7: Sitting upright

Whatever position you choose, you will need the support of your birthing partner, so do practise alternatives at home so you are familiar with the choices when the time comes. You will need to relax between the contractions of the second stage. So practise relaxing quickly to allow your body to recover between the bouts of hard work. When you are pushing, you need to make the most of each contraction and be guided by your body. Even if you have the desire to push, it may take a few contractions for you to get into the swing of things. At first it may feel just as though you are very constipated, due to the pressure on your bowel, but once baby has negotiated the curve of the pelvis and its head is under the symphysis pubis, you will feel the pressure stretching your perineum. Your midwife will be with you all the time in the second stage and will give you guidance and reassurance and tell you when to push. Push as you would to empty your bowels. You will probably find that you take a breath in but it should not be an enormous one and don't hold it for too long as this could affect the blood supply to baby. Breathe out as you begin to feel uncomfortable. You may need to bear down four or five times during each contraction. Listen to your midwife – she will guide you through.

When baby's head is stretching the skin at the perineum, it causes a painful sensation rather like putting your little fingers in the corners of your mouth and pulling your fingers apart. Imagine a roundish head stretching all diameters of your perineum. This is called **crowning**. Your midwife will ask you to stop pushing. This is to give her time to control the delivery of baby's head as well as allowing the perineum to stretch gradually. She will ask you to pant for a few seconds before pushing again, then pant again, push again and alternate until your baby's head has been born. The midwife will check that the umbilical cord is not round baby's neck, wipe the eyes and clean the nose and mouth. A further contraction will deliver baby's body – you may have to alternate panting and pushing again to help control delivery of the shoulders, but then your baby will be born.

Third stage

The third stage will take approximately five minutes and the placenta will be delivered. You may be asked to give a cough or a gentle push as the placenta is expelled by one last contraction. This will be painless and you might not even notice that the placenta is delivered if you are preoccupied with your baby.

Role of the birthing partner

Your partner can play a very important role in the birth of your baby but only if both of you wish him to be present. No one should be forced into a situation where they are not totally happy because they feel it is expected of them. Neither should you feel you must have a companion if you would rather not.

Most delivery suites welcome a labour companion of either sex, but women who are in a stable relationship usually choose their partner. Apart from being a familiar face and an emotional and physical support, your birthing partner can be responsible for various tasks which will not only help you but will also assist the staff if they are busy.

Ideally your birthing partner will have attended at least one joint antenatal session on labour, better still a whole course, so he can reinforce the coping skills you learnt at the classes and remind you of your breathing and relaxation techniques and comfortable positions. Your partner may even breathe in time with you during your contractions and is the ideal person to recognize if you start to tense or panic-breathe. He can reinforce instructions from your midwife and remind you of the milestones reached along the way. It is very comforting to have a close supporter with whom you can completely relax and share doubts and worries. You will also enjoy the physical reassurance that close contact can bring. This may take the form of merely holding hands, stroking or massage.

Your partner can be the one to help you to get into the different positions you have practised together and give you moral and physical support as your labour progresses. Between the contractions, he can stretch or massage your legs if you get cramp and wipe your face and neck with a cool damp flannel if you get too warm. The presence of your partner giving active support at the birth of your baby is the start of a new family life which both of you will share right from the beginning.

Rehearsal of labour

You may find it helpful to practice your breathing and relaxation through a few imaginary contractions which your partner can time for you. This is sometimes called a rehearsal of labour and you may have gone through this at your antenatal classes. Ask your partner to talk you through contractions of varying lengths and remind you how to breathe at the various stages.

Early first stage

You may feel the very early contractions as slight backache or period pains but they are more uncomfortable than painful. They may last up to 40 seconds and may be up to 30 minutes apart. If it is night-time try to rest, but during the day you may prefer to carry on the everyday activities, have a light snack, relax in a warm bath or pass the time watching television.

First stage contractions

The contractions are now stronger and you may describe them as very uncomfortable or even painful. They may last 50–60 seconds and be 5–10 minutes apart. You may wish to remain active but concentrate on each contraction as it comes. Now is the time to put your five point plan into action.

The contraction is starting now:
* greet the contraction positively and sigh out;
* check that you are in a comfortable position;
* check that your shoulders and hands are relaxed;
* breathe low and slow and concentrate on the outward breath. As the contraction rises to a peak and stays there, continue to breathe easily throughout, don't tense up.

The contraction is beginning to die away:
* give a sigh of relief at the end and check you are relaxed.

Later first stage contractions

By now the contractions will be very strong, may last about 60–90 seconds and be only two to three minutes apart. You may have had some form of pain relief and prefer to be less active. The contraction will be at its peak for about 45 seconds and you will feel as though it is taking over your whole body – let it, don't try to resist or fight it.

Your 'five point plan' still holds good but you may need to concentrate on **S**ighing **O**ut **S**lowly during the contraction. Stay relaxed and don't forget the long sigh at the end.

End of first stage

This is a transitional stage before the uterus starts to push the baby down the birth canal. The contractions now are very powerful, will last up to 90 seconds and may be every two minutes. You have been working very hard and will feel emotionally and physically drained. You may think that you cannot carry on any longer, you may even turn on your partner and tell him to go. These are recognizable reactions at this time and mean that it won't be much longer before you are in the second stage.

You may feel or be sick and there may be pressure on your back passage which makes you want to push at the peak of the contraction. *Never push* until your midwife has confirmed that you are in the second stage. There may be a few contractions where you need to stop yourself from pushing. Roll on to your side or into the kneeling position with your head on your forearms, and use the 'breathing-in-threes' (puff-puff-blow) technique to help you through the contractions. At the end of these you deserve two sighs of relief!

Second stage contractions

Sometimes the contractions diminish for a short time after full dilatation of the cervix. You can make the most of this short rest by relaxing. When the contractions return you will probably feel as though you want to bear down with them, but there is no need to push unless you have the urge to do so. When you are pushing, adopt your chosen position and bear down steadily, remembering not to hold your breath for more than a few seconds. You may need four or five pushes with each contraction. Relax completely between contractions and breathe slowly and deeply. Gradually you will feel the pressure of your baby's head stretching your perineum. Try not to tighten your pelvic floor during the contractions.

Crowning

As baby's head is stretching the perineum to its limit, you will feel a tight, burning sensation. Stay calm and listen to your midwife. She will tell you to stop pushing and to pant deeply just for a few seconds, then to push, perhaps to pant again and then push again. This will allow your baby's head to be born slowly. During the next contraction you may be asked to pant again as the shoulders are delivered, the rest of the baby will slide out easily.

At last the hard work is over – 'Congratulations!'

Using coping skills with conventional pain relief

Epidural

Even if you plan to have an epidural, the coping skills you have learnt can be used early on in your labour. They will also help when the epidural is being set up and when it needs topping up.

Pethidine

This may make you drowsy, so your birthing partner will have to play a more active role talking you through your 'five point plan'.

Entonox (gas and air)

Your midwife will show you how to use the entonox. Your partner will need to remind you to relax your shoulders and jawline especially when you are using the mouthpiece.

TENS

TENS stands for transcutaneous electric nerve stimulation and is a small battery-operated unit which you can control. It will take some of the pain of the contractions away and will allow you to use all your coping skills and to change your position frequently.

TENS should be applied early in labour and if the contractions become very painful, pethidine and/or entonox can be used as well as TENS. A combination of pain relief is often more effective than just one form. Your midwife will give you details of how to hire a unit if your delivery suite does not supply a service.

SECTION THREE

After the Birth

If you have recently delivered, you will be experiencing very different and changing emotions: exhilaration, triumph, perhaps deflation, and you will probably be feeling exhausted and ready for a well-earned rest. However, it is important to try out some simple exercises soon after your baby's birth.

The following pages explain the exercises you can safely start straight after vaginal delivery and continue for up to two weeks afterwards. If you have had a Caesarean delivery there is a special section for you on p.49.

Later on, there are further exercises for you to perform up to three months after birth.

From the day of delivery
Circulatory exercises

You will be resting more than usual over the next few days, so you need to maintain or improve your circulation by doing brisk foot and leg exercises several times whenever you think about it.

FOOT EXERCISES

Lie with your legs straight.

- Bend and stretch your ankles briskly for at least half a minute.
- Keeping your knees and hips still, circle both feet in as large a circle as you can for at least half a minute, changing direction halfway.

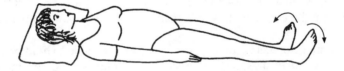

Fig. 3.1: Foot-circling exercise

LEG TIGHTENING

Lie or sit on the bed with your legs supported and straight.

- Pull both feet upwards at the ankle and press the back of your knees down on to the bed. Hold this position while you count to four, then relax. Repeat 12 times.

Remember to breathe normally whilst you do these exercises!

Breathing

A few deep breaths after you have finished your foot and leg exercises should also help your circulation as well as expanding your lungs fully now that your baby has moved out of the way. However, don't take more than three or four deep breaths at any one time or you may feel dizzy.

Pelvic floor

You may be feeling numb, or bruised and sore down below, especially if you have stitches. You may have had a forceps or other assisted delivery. Whatever type of delivery, your pelvic floor muscles need to be worked as soon as possible. These muscles form a hammock across the bottom of your pelvis and help to support the pelvic contents and control the openings of the three passages which run through them from your bladder, womb and bowel. If these muscles don't return to normal after the birth, you could suffer from stress incontinence – many women do. To help prevent problems, tone up the pelvic floor muscles by exercising your pelvic floor as often as possible for at least six weeks after your baby's birth, and then occasionally for the rest of your life. This should improve your sex life too.

Choose a comfortable position in which to do the exercise. If you find you are sore whilst exercising when sitting or lying on your back, try lying on your side or your front, relaxing in a warm bath, or even standing up. Practising pelvic floor contractions will help your wound to heal and feel less sore.

PELVIC FLOOR EXERCISE

Remember, you can do this exercise in any position you find comfortable but don't cross your legs.

*   Close your back passage as though you were stopping wind, close your middle and front passages too as though stopping the flow of urine. Squeeze and lift up all three passages inside. Hold strongly for as long as you can up to ten seconds, breathing normally throughout. Relax slowly and rest for a few seconds. Repeat the exercise **slowly** as many times as you can up to a maximum of ten.

At first you may not feel much happen, or may not be able to hold on to the tightening – don't worry, the exercise will get easier as you practise and become less sore. When you feel confident with the slow tightening, repeat the pelvic floor exercise lifting and letting go **more quickly** up to ten times.

Both the slow and the quicker pelvic-floor exercises can be done whilst you are doing things for your baby, for example, feeding, bathing, washing. You could practise whilst sitting on the lavatory **after** each bladder-emptying. This is a relaxed position in which to contract these muscles. Put a sticky coloured dot on the bathroom door and elsewhere around the house to remind you.

To prevent any leakage of urine, try to brace (tighten) your pelvic floor muscles **before** you cough, sneeze, laugh, or lift something. Sometimes it takes three months or more before your pelvic floor is back to normal and it is advisable to test its strength **before** resuming strenuous physical activities (see pelvic floor stress test, p.60).

Rest and relaxation

Get as much rest as you can in the early days and try to catch up on lost sleep, particularly if you laboured during the night. Use your relaxation technique to help you to get off to sleep. Remember that you can lie on your tummy again now, unless you have had a Caesarean birth. This is a very comfortable position in which to rest especially if the area where your stitches are is feeling bruised and sore, or if the bottom of your spine is painful. Try placing a couple of pillows under your hips and another under your head and hopefully you will drop off for a much-needed sleep.

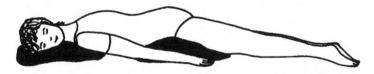

Fig. 3.2: Lying on front with pillows under hips

Try to get as much sleep and rest as you can in hospital before you go home.

To get out of bed, bend your knees up and keep them together. Pull in your tummy, roll on to your side keeping your knees and shoulders in line. Push up into a sitting position using your upper hand and lower elbow. Sit on the side of the bed for a moment. Stand up slowly straightening your legs. Do this in reverse or crawl forwards when getting into bed.

From the day after delivery

Keep up with your foot and leg exercises especially if your feet are swollen or the room is warm. Avoid standing unless you have to. Before you do a task, ask yourself if it is necessary to stand, or could you do it sitting down instead. If you had a general anaesthetic during your delivery, continue to do the deep breathing exercises.

Abdominal exercises

Your tummy may feel like a blancmange and doesn't look as though it will ever fit into your jeans again! If you didn't put on too much weight during your pregnancy, the muscles are probably just stretched. By the end of a first pregnancy the long muscles of the abdomen – the recti – can stretch to about two-thirds longer than their original length. In subsequent pregnancies, these muscles may even double in length.

It is quite safe to try the following two abdominal exercises on the day after your baby is delivered or on the same day, if you are feeling up to it.

TUMMY-TIGHTENING

Lie on your back with one pillow under your head, your knees bent up and your feet flat on the bed.

- Breathe in, breathe out, tighten your tummy muscles and pull the lower part of your tummy in towards your spine. Hold whilst you count up to four, breathing normally throughout. Repeat up to ten times, gradually increasing the length of time you hold your tummy in up to a count of ten.

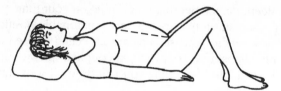

Fig. 3.3: Tummy tightening in lying

This is a very simple exercise for your abdominal muscles but a very important one. It can be performed frequently in any position such as sitting or standing (and later on, whilst kneeling on all-fours).. Try to get into the habit of practising it when you are feeding your baby or having a drink. You can progress the time you hold the tightening up to a count of ten when you feel able, so that after a couple of weeks, you may be doing ten tightenings and holding for ten seconds several times a day in different positions.

The pelvic tilting exercise you performed during pregnancy is also one to use now. It will help to reduce the length of the rectus muscles so allowing them to regain their former strength and function.

PELVIC TILTING

Lie on your back with one pillow under your head, your knees bent up and put your feet flat on the bed.

- Pull in your tummy muscles, tighten the muscles of your buttocks and press the small of your back down on to the bed. Hold this position whilst you count to four, breathing normally, then relax. Repeat at least five times.

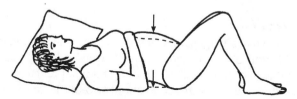

Fig. 3.4: Pelvic tilting in lying

The exercise may also be performed more rhythmically to help relieve any backache you may have following delivery. Gradually increase the number of repetitions to ten or more over the next couple of weeks. Try pelvic tilting in other positions too, for instance, sitting and standing may be more convenient than lying when you are at home and time is precious.

PELVIC TILTING IN SITTING

Sit well back on a dining-type chair with your hands resting on your knees and your feet flat on the floor.

- Pull in your tummy muscles, tighten your buttock muscles and press the small of your back into the back of the chair. Hold for a count of four, breathing normally, then relax. Repeat five times, progressing to ten times or more.

PELVIC TILTING IN STANDING
Stand tall with your feet a few inches apart and knees slightly bent.

- Imagine you are zipping up your jeans! Pull in your tummy muscles and tighten your buttocks. Hold for a count of four, breathing normally, then relax. Repeat five times, progressing to ten times or more.

As with your pelvic-floor exercise, pelvic tilting can be performed in many positions whilst you are carrying out many activities like feeding your baby, washing up, having a bath. It is particularly important to practise your pelvic tilting when standing (sideways in front of a mirror if possible) to check your posture. You are not pregnant any longer, but your body may need to be reminded of this fact. So always stand tall with your tummy and bottom tucked in and your shoulders down and relaxed.

Further abdominal exercises from the third day

Note that before doing further abdominal exercises you should check that your rectus muscles are realigning and that there is no undue gap between them (diastasis of the recti). If you start to do stronger exercises or work the oblique muscles when you have a gap, the distance between the recti may widen further. This is because the oblique and transverse muscles are inserted into the linea alba (see p.3) and the exercise may pull and increase the gap.

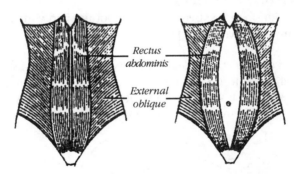

Rectus abdominis

External oblique

Fig. 3.5: Diastasis of recti postpartum

Up to two fingers width between the rectus muscles is considered acceptable from two to three days after delivery but, if your gap is greater than this, rotation and other abdominal exercises should not be performed to avoid the risk of any increase in the separation. You can check your own muscles to assess the gap, or you can ask your partner or midwife to do it for you. The best time to do the 'rec check' is from the third day following delivery.

SELF 'REC-CHECK' FOR DIASTASIS RECTI

Lie on your back with one pillow under your head; bend your knees up and put your feet flat on the bed. Place two fingers into your abdomen just below your umbilicus (navel) with the palm of your hand facing you. Pull in your tummy, then lift your head and shoulders forwards towards your knees and you should feel your rectus muscles pressing against the sides of your fingers as you lift. Lower your head down slowly. Breathe normally throughout.

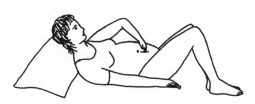

Fig. 3.6: Self-check for diastasis recti

At this stage, a gap of two fingers width is acceptable and you may progress to the further abdominal exercises described later. If the gap is much wider and you can fit three or even four fingers between your recti, do not progress to the further exercises just yet. Instead, there are special exercises for you to do in order to help close this gap to an acceptable width (see p. 62).

Add the following abdominal exercises to your programme after you've done your 'rec-check' and the gap is two fingers width or less.

The exercises will be more effective if performed slowly and the number of repetitions increased according to your individual capability. It is always better to exercise little and often rather than just once a day. However, if you are feeling tired or unwell, be guided by your body and leave the exercises until you are feeling better.

Hip-hitching (waist trimmer)

Lie on your back with one knee bent and your foot flat and your other leg straight. Place one hand on your waist above your straight leg.

• Slide the heel of your straight leg down, away from your waist, so that your leg becomes longer. Pull in your tummy muscles and shorten the same leg by drawing your hip up towards your ribs at that side, keeping your knee straight. Hold, then relax. Do this exercise six times with each leg.

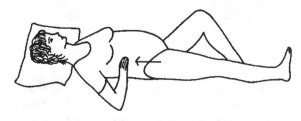

Fig. 3.7: Hip-hitching in lying

Gradually increase the number of repetitions to 12 or more each side over the following weeks.

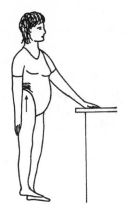

Try hip-hitching in standing if it is more convenient to do so during the day.

Stand with your feet a little way apart, holding on to a firm support, e.g. a work surface, table, bannister.

- Pull in your tummy muscles and shorten one leg by drawing your hip up towards your ribs at one side, keeping your knee straight. Hold, then lower the leg down on to the floor. Do this exercise six times with each leg.

You can increase the number of repetitions to 12 or more to each side by about six weeks after delivery.

Fig. 3.8: Hip-hitching in standing

Straight curl-up (tummy flattener)

Lie on your back with one pillow under your head and with your hands on the front of your thighs. Bend your knees up and put your feet flat.

- Pull in your tummy muscles, tighten the muscles of your buttocks and press the small of your back down on to the support (pelvic tilt). Hold this position whilst lifting your head and shoulders forwards, sliding your hands towards your knees. Breathe normally, then slowly lower your head and shoulders back down on to the pillow before relaxing your pelvic tilt. Repeat five times.

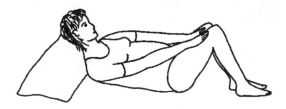

Fig. 3.9: Straight curl-up

Gradually increase the number of repetitions to 12 or more over the following weeks. Have a rest half way through if you need it. **Always** bend your knees whilst performing this exercise and tilt your pelvis before lifting your head and shoulders to protect your back.

Note that your abdomen must stay flat throughout the straight and oblique curl-up exercises; if there is any 'peaking or doming', this is an indication that the recti could still be separated, so only curl to the point just before this occurs. Progress to the following abdominal exercises when you can hold your abdomen flat.

Oblique curl-up (tummy and waist trimmer)

Lie on your back with one pillow under your head and your arms by your side. Bend your knees up and put your feet flat.

- Pull in your tummy muscles, tighten the muscles of your buttocks and press the small of your back down on to the support (pelvic tilt). Hold this position whilst lifting your head and shoulders forwards, reaching with your left hand in the direction of your right ankle whilst breathing normally (your hand may only reach the outside of the opposite knee). Slowly lower down to the pillow and relax your tummy muscles completely. Change to reaching to the left side with your right hand. Repeat five times to each side.

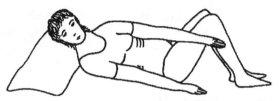

Fig. 3.10: Oblique curl-up

Gradually increase the number of repetitions to 12 or more each side over the following weeks. Have a rest half way if you need to. You can also increase the difficulty of the previous two exercises as your muscles get stronger by removing the pillow from under your head.

Knee-rolling (tummy and waist trimmer)

Lie on your back with one pillow under your head and your arms out to the side. Bend your knees up and put your feet flat.

- Pull in your tummy muscles, tighten the muscles of your buttocks and press the small of your back down on to the support (pelvic tilt). Keep your knees together and slowly roll both knees over to your left as far as possible, keeping your shoulders flat. Return your knees to the centre and relax your tummy muscles. Pelvic tilt again and repeat the exercise slowly to your right side before returning your knees to the centre and relaxing. Repeat the exercise five times to each side.

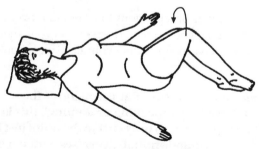

Fig. 3.11: Knee-rolling

Gradually increase the number of repetitions to 12 or more each side over the following weeks. You should be able to take your knees further towards the floor as your muscles strengthen.

Postnatal exercises and care following caesarean delivery

If you have had a Caesarean birth you will need extra rest but exercises are still important, even on your first day.

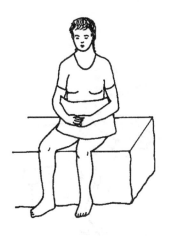

Fig. 3.12: Supported coughing

Your circulation will be much slower after a Caesarean delivery and so vigorous **foot and leg** exercises should be performed especially if you had epidural anaesthesia. Taking two or three **deep breaths** regularly whilst you are relatively immobile will help to improve the ventilation of your chest.

If you had a general anaesthetic, you may feel you want to cough. Take a few deep breaths in and out then 'huff' (a short forced breath out) and this will help to loosen any secretions that may be present. Before you cough, bend your knees up and support your stitches with your hands or a pillow, whilst leaning forwards. This will be more comfortable and prevent undue strain on your stitches.

Flatulence or wind is often the cause of great discomfort after a Caesarean delivery and may be relieved by bending your knees and gently rocking them a few inches from side to side.

Note that the knees should not be taken any further to the sides in case any diastasis of recti is present.

The easiest and safest way of moving up and down the bed is by bending your knees, pulling in your tummy and curling forwards whilst pushing on your hands and feet. You will be able to move your body in a forwards or backwards direction. Don't attempt to sit up forwards from a lying position, but instead roll over on to your side and push yourself up into a sitting position using your arms.

Getting out of bed

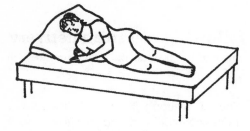

- bend your knees up and keep them together;
- pull your tummy in;
- roll your whole body over to one side – don't twist;

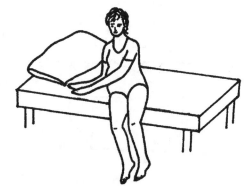

- push up into a sitting position using your upper hand and lower elbow, swinging your legs now over the side of the bed;

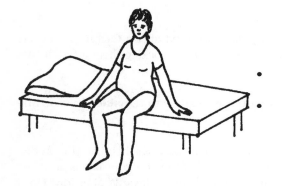

- sit on the side of the bed for a moment;
- stand up slowly, straightening your legs.

Do this in reverse when getting into bed.

Fig. 3.13: Getting out of bed

When you are standing and walking you may be inclined to lean forwards to protect your wound. Do try to stand up straight and walk tall to prevent backache.

Pelvic-floor exercises are still important to do even if you have had a Caesarean birth, as the hormones and the weight of your baby put extra stress on these muscles during pregnancy. If you have a catheter in place, only try an occasional tightening before it is removed.

Tummy-tightening and **pelvic tilting** can also be started from your first day. If you do pelvic tilting rhythmically, it helps to relieve any backache which might have been caused by the tilted position necessary for your operation, or by tension in your back muscles following an epidural. A check for diastasis of the recti can be done whenever you feel comfortable, probably around the fifth day. If the gap is less than two fingers width, then move on to the further abdominal exercises suggested for a vaginal delivery but progress slowly (see p.45).

You will need more rest and support at home after what is really major surgery as well as giving birth. When you start driving again depends on your rate of recovery as you must be able to concentrate fully and perform an emergency stop. You will also need to check with your insurance company regarding their policy before this.

The following advice is for all mothers - whatever type of delivery.

Care of your back

During the early postnatal period your joints are still unstable because of the hormonal influence on the ligaments causing them to remain lax for up to six months, or even longer if you are still breastfeeding. Your abdominal muscles, which normally help to support the spine and control the pelvic tilt, have been stretched and are weak. So your back is more vulnerable and ideally you should not be doing tasks which involve bending, stooping or lifting. Unfortunately your baby's needs will involve lots of these activities and you won't be able to delegate them all!

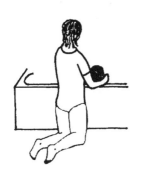

Fig. 3.14: Bathing baby

Before doing any tasks for baby, stop and think if you could do them in a more comfortable position and so put less stress and strain on your body. Discuss positions for changing and bathing your baby which avoid stooping and carrying heavy baths of water.

Could you stand at a surface which is at waist height, or kneel at a surface which is coffee-table height which would remove the need for stooping whilst carrying out tasks such as changing your baby's nappy. Perhaps you could place the baby's bath inside the family bath and kneel to avoid bending over. You would also avoid having to lift the baby bath full of water.

Try to carry objects, such as baby carry seats, close to your body. Carrying on one side only puts a strain on your joints and muscles. Remind your partner about this too.

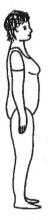

Posture

Correct posture in all positions will not only ease backache, but should also give you a sense of good body-image. At first, it will be a matter of re-educating your posture in front of a full-length mirror as your body has got used to the pregnant stance. If you stand sideways to the mirror you will soon see whether your outline is still a semi-pregnant one! Check your posture whenever you stand up, it will soon become a good habit.

Fig. 3.15: Posture in standing

Feeding baby should be a relaxed and happy time for both of you. Make sure you are in a comfortable and supported position. If you choose sitting try resting your baby on a pillow to avoid aching in your shoulders and back from leaning forwards.

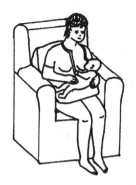

If you have stitches you may be more comfortable lying on your side to breast or bottlefeed or sitting on pillows.

Fig. 3.16: Position for feeding

Lifting

Lifting must be kept to an absolute minimum for the first few weeks if this is at all possible. This is the advice that would be given to a patient who was already complaining of back problems, but it is also important to try to prevent problems occurring in the first place. Of course you may have to lift if there is no one else to do it for you. In that case make sure the object handled is as light as possible and hold it close to your body.

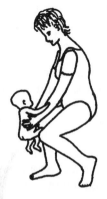

Fig. 3.17: Correct lifting

With a little planning, perhaps you can delegate some lifting to others but, if you have no help, follow the correct lifting procedures as described on p.16 to avoid back strain at this very vulnerable time.

If you have toddlers, let them climb up on to your knee or a chair instead of being lifted, or on to the second or third stair for dressing so you can avoid stooping. Alternatively you could kneel on the floor.

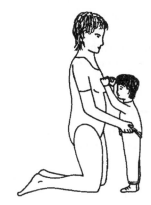

Fig. 3.18: Dressing toddler

Daily activities

Leave heavy housework, such as vacuuming, moving furniture and cleaning windows for as long as possible unless you can delegate these jobs. All of these tasks put a strain on your back. Walking is a good way of supplementing your postnatal exercises but don't forget you always have to get back to base so don't go too far to start with! Get help with the heavy shopping.

Rest and relaxation at home

When you go home, there are extra demands on you at a time when hormonal changes are going on and you are feeling tired and emotional. Plenty of rest will help you to cope better.

Try to make sure you have an afternoon sleep for the next few weeks. If you have had a broken night with baby, try to lie-in the following morning until the next feed is due. Remember your relaxation techniques. These will help you and your partner to sleep better and relieve tension caused by the many worries and anxieties a new baby brings. Just a short spell of relaxation will help to revitalize you!

Exercises after two weeks

Continue to follow your previous programme of exercises and advice. However, at this stage you should be much less sore and, if you are feeling ready, you may start some additional exercises to help you to get your figure back into shape. You will need a firm surface like the floor to lie on for most of the exercises, but some can be done sitting or standing. As you get used to doing the exercises, you may want to increase the number of times you repeat them up to about 12 times.

Side-bending on all-fours (waist trimmer)

Kneel on all-fours, with your hands directly under your shoulders and your knees directly under your hips – arms and thighs vertical and your back level, not hollow.

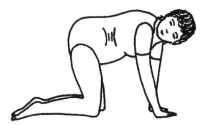

- Pull up your tummy muscles, move your head and right shoulder round towards your right hip, at the same time bend your right hip towards your right shoulder. Return to midline, then bend to the left side. Repeat five times to each side.

Fig. 3.19: Side-bending on all-fours

Hip extension lying on your front (buttock toner)

Lie on your front without a pillow and your arms down by your side.

- Lift your left leg keeping your knee straight and the front of your left hip in contact with the floor. Hold, then slowly lower your leg back down to the floor. Repeat five times with each leg, breathing normally throughout.

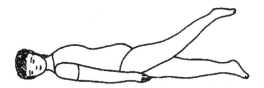

Fig. 3.20: Hip extension

Pelvic tilting on all-fours (tummy flattener)

Kneel on all-fours, with your hands directly under your shoulders and your knees directly under your hips – arms and thighs vertical.

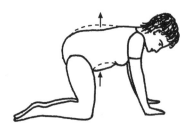

- Pull up your tummy muscles and push the small of your back up towards the ceiling. Breathe normally, then relax slowly allowing your back to flatten – **not hollow**. Repeat five times slowly.

Fig. 3.21: Pelvic tilting on all-fours

Side-bending lying on your back (waist trimmer)

Lie on your back without a pillow and with your knees bent and your arms by your side.

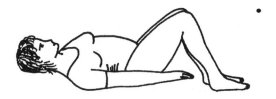

Fig. 3.22: Side-bending in back lying

- Pull in your tummy muscles, lift your head slightly and slide your right hand down the outside of your right leg towards your ankle. Return to the centre and relax slowly. Repeat five times to each side breathing normally throughout.

Side-bending in sitting (waist trimmer)

Sit well back on a stool or on the edge of the bed with your feet firmly on the floor.

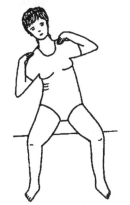

Fig. 3.23: Side-bending in sitting

- Rest your fingers on your shoulders. Pull in your tummy muscles and bend sideways at your waist so your right elbow is nearly touching the outside of your right hip. Do not lean forwards or allow your hips to lift from the support. Straighten up to the centre, relax your tummy muscles, then repeat to the left. Repeat five times to each side.

Shoulder circling in sitting (to relieve tension)

Sit well back on a stool or on the edge of the bed, with your feet firmly on the floor.

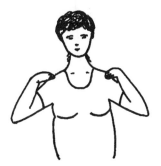

- Rest your fingers on your shoulders. Slowly and rhythmically make large backward circles with your elbows. Repeat five times.

Fig. 3.24: Shoulder circling in sitting

Twisting in sitting (tummy and waist trimmer)
Sit well back on a stool or on the edge of the bed with your feet firmly on the floor.

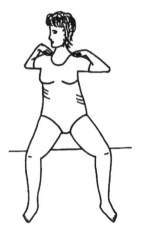

- Rest your fingers on your shoulders and lift your elbows sideways in line with your shoulders. Pull in your tummy muscles and twist the upper part of your body round to the right as far as possible from the waist, keeping your hips down and your back upright. Return to the midline, then twist to the left. Repeat five times to each side.

Fig. 3.25: Twisting in sitting

Side-bends in standing (waist trimmer)
Stand with your feet apart and your arms by your sides.

- Pull in your tummy muscles and slide the fingers of your right hand down the outside of your right thigh as far as possible without leaning forwards. Return to midline and relax your tummy muscles. Repeat to the left with your left arm. Repeat five times to each side.

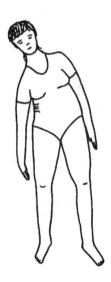

Fig. 3.26: Side-bending in standing

Twisting in standing (tummy and waist trimmer)

Stand with your feet apart and your arms out to the sides at shoulder level.

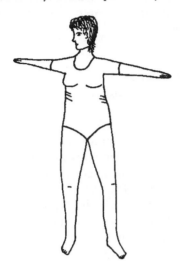

- Pull in your tummy muscles and twist your head and upper part of your body and arms round to the right as far as possible from the waist, keeping your hips facing forwards, your arms back and your back upright. Return to the midline, then twist to the left. Repeat five times to each side.

Fig. 3.27: Twisting in standing

Exercises to avoid

Two commonly-practised 'abdominal' exercises are double-leg raising and sit-ups with straight legs. These are very high-risk exercises for anyone to perform and may result in compression injury to vertebral discs or muscle and ligament damage. They are even more risky when you have been pregnant because of your stretched muscles and lax ligaments.

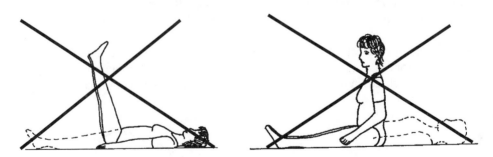

Fig. 3.28: Double-leg raising and sit-ups with straight legs

These two exercises should never be performed

Exercises after six weeks

Still continue to practice your previous exercises especially those for your pelvic floor (do the stress test in a few weeks, see p.60). Continue to follow the advice on back care and rest. If you feel ready, you can now add some stronger exercises in preparation for returning to more strenuous exercise and sport.

Stronger straight curl-up (tummy flattener)

Lie on your back without a pillow and your arms folded across your chest. Bend your knees up and put your feet flat.

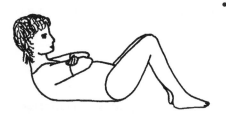

Fig. 3.29: Straight curl-up

- Pull in your tummy muscles, tighten the muscles of your buttocks and press the small of your back down on to the support (pelvic tilt). Hold this position whilst lifting your head and shoulders forwards. Breathe normally, then slowly lower your head and shoulders back down before relaxing your pelvic tilt. Repeat five times.

Gradually increase the number of repetitions to 12 or more over the following weeks. Have a rest half way through if you need it. **Always** bend your knees whilst performing this exercise and tilt your pelvis before lifting your head and shoulders. Remember to keep your tummy flat.

Back extension (for your buttocks and back)

Lie on your front without a pillow and your arms down by your side.

- Tighten your buttocks and lift both your legs keeping your knees straight and the front of your hips in contact with the floor. Hold, then slowly lower your legs back down to the floor. Repeat five times, breathing normally throughout.

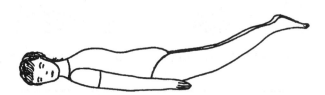

Fig. 3.30: Back extension

You can increase the number of repetitions to 12 or more over the next few weeks, resting halfway if you need to.

Stronger knee-rolling (tummy and waist trimmer)

Lie on your back with your arms out to the side. Bend your knees up and put your feet flat.

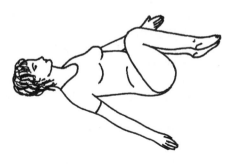

Fig. 3.31: Stronger knee-rolling

- Pull in your tummy muscles and bend both of your knees up on to your chest. Keep your tummy pulled in and roll both knees over to the floor on your left, keeping your shoulders flat. Return your knees to the centre and relax your tummy muscles. Pull in your tummy again and repeat the exercise to your right side. Repeat the exercise five times to each side.

You can increase the number of repetitions to 12 or more to each side over the next few weeks, resting halfway if you feel you need to.

Leg-lifting (thigh toner)

Lie on one side with your underneath leg bent, and your head resting on your underneath hand.

- Pull in your tummy muscles and lift your top leg up sideways in line with your body, keeping your knee straight. Hold, then lower down slowly. Do five more lifts, then roll over on to your other side and repeat with the other leg.

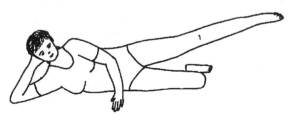

Fig. 3.32: Leg-lifting

Gradually increase the number of repetitions up to 12 with a rest halfway if you need to.

Stronger oblique curl-up (waist and tummy trimmer)

Lie on your back without a pillow and your hands one on each side of your head. Bend your knees up and put your feet flat.

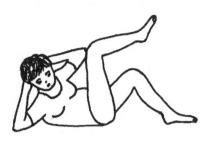

Fig. 3.33: Stronger oblique curl-up

- Pull in your tummy muscles, tighten the muscles of your buttocks and press the small of your back down on to the floor (pelvic tilt). Keeping your back flat, lift your head and left shoulder and your right knee off the floor so that your left elbow and right knee touch. Hold for a few seconds then return to the starting position slowly and relax your tummy muscles. Repeat with the opposite elbow and knee. Start with five repetitions and gradually build up to 12 or more over the next few weeks with a rest halfway if you need to.

Pelvic floor stress test

You can test the strength of your pelvic floor about 10–12 weeks after your baby's birth and before returning to strenuous exercise and sport. Jump up and down with a full bladder and cough deeply two or three times while doing so.

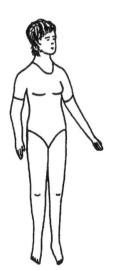

There should not be any leakage of urine if the muscles have regained their former strength and function. However if you do leak when testing, your pelvic-floor muscles will need further intensive exercising. Ask your doctor or health visitor to refer you to an obstetric physiotherapist for individual advice and treatment if required. You may be able to ring your physiotherapist directly. Another pregnancy could make your pelvic floor weaker, so ensure your muscles are strong again before deciding to have another baby.

Fig. 3.34: Stress test

Returning to strenuous exercise and sport

Strenuous keep-fit classes, aerobics or competitive sports should be left for at least 10–12 weeks and only resumed after you have passed the pelvic floor stress test. Even at this stage your joints may not yet be fully protected by your ligaments and so extra care is still needed. Back care, good posture and pelvic floor exercises are still a must for the rest of your life!

If you are beginning any new activity or sport, do start gently and build up gradually. If you were a regular exerciser, you will be able to progress more quickly but beware of overdoing things. Before this, you might like to join specially designed exercise-to-music or aquanatal classes which are often held locally. Make sure that they are run by personnel qualified to teach postnatal exercises. If you need any advice your obstetric physiotherapist, health visitor or ante/postnatal exercise teacher should be able to help you.

Some physical postnatal problems

Although you will receive help and support from your midwife and other health professionals in hospital and when you are at home, there may not be an obstetric physiotherapist in your area. These additional hints may be useful if you have any of the following physical problems postnatally.

Painful perineum

If you have a sore perineum, you may find it difficult to get into a comfortable position for feeding your baby. Try sitting with a pillow under each buttock to relieve the pressure on the perineum or lying on your side with a pillow between your knees. A very comfortable resting position is on your tummy with a pillow under your hips and another under your head and shoulders. Many mothers forget that they can lie on their tummies once more!

The pain can be eased considerably by the application of ice. This must be used with caution as it is possible to give yourself an ice-burn. Put some crushed ice or a packet of frozen peas in a polythene bag wrapped in a clean damp flannel to prevent contact with the skin. Place this over the painful area for **no longer than ten minutes** – a good position is lying on your side with a pillow between your knees. Never sit on the ice pack! Alternatively, the painful area can be massaged for **up to ten minutes** by an ice cube held in a disposable cloth as long as you keep the ice cube moving.

When the pain is easing, remember to practise your pelvic floor exercises as the rhythmical contraction and relaxation of your muscles will help to improve the local circulation.

Diastasis recti

If you have discovered a wide gap between your rectus muscles when you did your 'rec-check' (see p.46) you need to pay special attention to decreasing this gap. Remember your abdominal muscles help to support your back and if they are weak you may get backache now or suffer from back problems later in life.

SPECIAL EXERCISES FOR DIASTASIS RECTI

The easiest exercise which you can practise in any position is **tummy tightening.**

- Breathe in, breathe out, tighten your tummy muscles and pull the lower part of your tummy in towards your spine. Hold whilst you count up to four, breathing normally throughout. Repeat up to ten times, gradually increasing the length of time you hold your tummy in up to a count of ten.

You can do this in bed, in the bath, sitting feeding your baby, changing nappies, standing washing your hands. The more often you do it, the quicker you will get your muscles working more effectively. Aim to do ten tightenings, holding each for a count of ten, several times a day in different positions.

Also try the following exercises as often as you can.

PELVIC TILTING WITH HANDS ACROSS THE ABDOMEN

Lie on your back with one pillow under your head, your knees bent up and your feet flat on the bed. Place your hands overlapping across your abdomen.

- Pull in your tummy muscles, tighten the muscles of your buttocks and press the small of your back down on to the bed. At the same time, pull your rectus muscles towards midline with your hands, narrowing the gap between them. Hold this position whilst you count to four, breathing normally, then relax. Repeat five times.

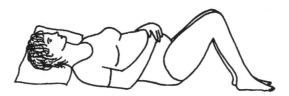

Fig. 3.35: Pelvic tilting with hands across abdomen

- As above but, in addition, lift your head (not shoulders) towards your knees. Do not allow any 'peaking or doming' of your tummy muscles. Hold this position whilst you count to four, breathing normally, then relax. Repeat five times.

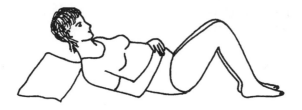

Fig. 3.36: Pelvic tilting with head lifting – hands across abdomen

Try to practise these exercises a few times each waking hour, increasing the number of repetitions gradually. Check the gap between your recti muscles once or twice a week until it has narrowed to two fingers width or less. Now it is safe to start the further abdominal exercises (see p.45).

Be extra careful getting out of bed. Roll over with your knees bent and together and push yourself up into a sitting position with your arms. If you try to sit up forwards, this could increase the gap between your muscles.

If there is a wide enough space to insert a fist between the muscles, ask your midwife to refer you to an obstetric physiotherapist for advice. It may be necessary to have some form of elasticated support for your abdominal muscles until the gap closes as well as practising the specific exercises above.

Diastasis symphysis pubis

You may have had this condition in late pregnancy due to hormonal influence. However, sometimes it occurs as a result of a difficult labour. Ideally you should be under the care of an obstetric physiotherapist. If you have a lot of pain postnatally, you need complete bed rest until the severe pain subsides. Whilst you are in bed it is especially important to perform your circulatory exercises and you can also practise pelvic floor exercises, tummy tightening and pelvic tilting. Do not attempt any further abdominal exercises until advised to do so.

You may be given a belt to support your pelvis but you must still be very careful how you move in bed. To turn over bend up both knees together, roll your body over keeping your knees pressed firmly together. Initially, ice may be used with caution as described for painful perineum, and may give you some relief of pain. As the pain eases and you start to get out of bed, follow this advice: bend both your knees up together, pull in your tummy, and roll on to your side pressing your knees firmly together and in line with your shoulders. Push up into a sitting position on the side of the bed using your upper hand and lower elbow. Sit on the side of the bed for a moment. Lower both of your feet to the floor at the same time and stand up slowly. Remember to do this sequence in reverse when you are getting back into bed to protect your symphysis. You may be offered a walking frame and may find it more comfortable to take small steps and wear your pelvic support when walking. Avoid stairs if at all possible. You will still need to be careful and protect your joint as you become more mobile, but the condition should gradually resolve.

Backache

You may have had backache antenatally, or it may have started since you delivered. Often it is postural due to the position you adopted during labour and made worse by looking after your baby. Remember your ligaments are still slack and your abdominal muscles weak and both these contribute to backache. Follow the back care and posture advice on pp.10 and 51. A hot water bottle wrapped in towels may help at home but if your back pain persists ask to be referred to an obstetric physiotherapist.

Coccydynia

Coccydynia (pain in the coccyx or tailbone) is usually caused by a difficult delivery and the advice on positions and ice for pain relief suggested for a painful perineum may help. Sit as upright as possible as this relieves the pressure on the coccyx. If the pain persists seek advice.

Urinary problems

The bladder may take some time to settle down after delivery. However, sometimes urinary problems persist especially if you had a forceps delivery. The main urinary problem postnatally is stress incontinence. This is when spurts of urine escape when you cough, laugh, sneeze, lift objects or perform sudden movements. Usually the main cause is weak pelvic floor muscles, so all women need to follow the pelvic floor programme (p.5) and to do the stress test (p.60). If after 10–12 weeks you still have a leakage problem, get a referral to an obstetric physiotherapist or gynaecologist.

Other urinary problems which sometimes appear postnatally are frequency and urgency. Frequency means that the woman feels she needs to empty her bladder very often. Urgency is when the woman has to dash to empty her bladder as soon as she feels she needs to. Both these problems can also be helped by specialist physiotherapy treatment.

Bowel problems

Bowel problems following delivery are much less common, but if faecal incontinence (leakage) persists, ask to be referred for specialist help.

Dyspareunia

Some women experience dyspareunia (painful intercourse) which can be very distressing. If this is a problem, try alternative positions and use lubricants, but if the pain persists ask your GP to refer you to a gynaecologist who may suggest physiotherapy.

Additional Information

Useful addresses

The Association of Chartered Physiotherapists in Women's Health (ACPWH)
c/o The Chartered Society of Physiotherapy
14 Bedford Row
London W1R 4ED
Tel: (0171) 306 6666

Diastasis Symphysis Pubis Help Group
c/o Pauline Best (London DSP Support Group)
20 Ashville Road
London E11 4DT
Tel: (0181) 558 3469

National Childbirth Trust (NCT)
Alexandra House
Oldham Terrace
London W3 6NH
Tel: (0181) 992 8637

Caesarean Support Group
Contact National Childbirth Trust (see above)

Videos

The BBC Pregnancy and Postnatal Exercise Video by ACPOG members. Available from: ACPWH Book Secretary, c/o The Chartered Society of Physiotherapy, 14 Bedford Row, London WC1R 4ED. Tel: (0171) 242 1941.

The Y Plan Before and After Pregnancy Video by YMCA. Available from: ACPWH Book Secretary, c/o The Chartered Society of Physiotherapy, 14 Bedford Row, London WC1R 4ED. Tel: (0171) 242 1941.